Fitness and Health

Introduction

I want to thank you and congratulate you for downloading the book, *"Health and Fitness"*.

This book has actionable information that will help you to live a healthy life.

According to a study conducted by Dr. Emanuele Di Angelantonio, from Cambridge University, unhealthy lifestyles like poor dieting and sedentary living have been seen to reduce your lifespan by up to 23 years! This means if you are 40 years old and you have been leading an unhealthy lifestyle, your life expectancy can drop from 78 years to just 55 years. Are you shocked? You should be.

You might not know this but when you make poor unhealthy eating choices and you don't keep fit, you expose your body to the possibility of attracting a wide range of excruciating consequences like getting heart diseases, diabetes, a stroke and cancer. Of course, no one wants to attract any of those diseases but we do because we don't have the knowledge on what to do to avoid them.

Lucky for you, in this book, you are going to be educated on how to be fit and healthy to a point that worrying about the above diseases will be a thing of the past for you. This book is going to provide you with a lifestyle formula that will not only enable you to live a long and healthy life but will also keep your body fit.

You are going to learn why health and fitness is important, what preparations you need to take to get started and what exercises you are supposed to do to get fit. You will also learn what foods you are supposed to eat to be healthy and to top it up, there is a 30 day meal plan that you can follow on your journey to a healthy living. Let's get started.

Thanks again for downloading this book. I hope you enjoy it!

Table of Contents

To give you the motivation to want to do something NOW, let's start by building an understanding of why you should care about being healthy and fit.

Why Is Being Healthy And Fit Important?

Thousands of years ago, human beings used to depend on hunting and gathering as their only source of food. Back then, everyone had a role to play in the community. Men used to hunt for food while women were responsible for tilling the land and gathering vegetables for cooking. Because of the physicality of the activities that humans undertook back then and their healthy diet which composed of natural foods that were free from any chemicals, things like diseases, which we see currently e.g. diabetes, cancer, heart disease and others, were a rare occurrence to them. They were both physically fit and healthy. This made them live longer as compared to the life expectancy that people have in the world today.

The story of how ancient men were fit and healthy normally sounds like an unreal story. This is because our era and their era are so different that it is even hard to imagine how they lived. Imagine a world with minimal to no diseases? It's definitely nothing like the world we know today.

So what happened? How did we get from being that healthy to being so unhealthy?

What happened is a question that will be answered by the events that occurred between the year 1760 to 1820. Around the year 1760, the world went through an industrial revolution. In this transition, different industries came up including factories which started manufacturing and processing foods for the purpose of giving foods a longer shelf life. The revolution also gave birth to technology innovation that saw human beings going from using hand production methods to using machines. After the industrialization revolution, the world as humans knew it back then changed completely. Among the things that changed, there were two things which immediately started affecting the health of human beings.

- The first thing was the reduction of physical activities. The physicality that human beings used in carrying out activities was reduced immensely by the introduction of machines. People started being less and less fit, which gave way to the emerging of various health problems like obesity and heart problems, which were diseases that were unheard of in the past.

- The second thing that happened is that the food that human beings were used to eat was not altered with chemicals, which posed a danger to their health. The birth of the food industries saw an emerging culture of people being convinced that processed food is better than natural foods and the industries encouraged that through adding sweeteners and chemicals that improved the shelf life of foods. As a result of that, people started getting strange diseases like cancer, diabetes and high blood pressure.

So why should the subject of health and fitness be important to you?

The answer lies in the two aforementioned points discussed above, which clearly indicate that the world is not what it used to be. Back in the days, health and fitness was not even a subject to be discussed because the environment and lifestyle encouraged people to unconsciously lead healthy and fit lives. But today, the subject of health and fitness is important because the world has provided us with an environment that encourages us to be unfit and unhealthy. An environment that makes us sit down in offices the whole day in the name of working and provides us with foods that have been infiltrated by chemicals and other additives, which are unhealthy to our bodies. We are living in a world where your health is in danger from the time that you are born and that's why the subject of health and fitness is important. Without the subject of health and fitness, it is impossible for you to acquire an athletic body and optimum health, which you desperately desire.

The answer to your health and fitness problems can only be solved by one thing and that's a lifestyle formula that illustrates how to live a healthy and fit life.

But What Can You Get Out Of Following A Healthy And Fit Lifestyle?

By learning and following a healthy and fit lifestyle, you will be able to not only gain a nice body shape but also a body which is energetic and healthy. But that's not all; there are also other benefits that you will stand to gain as explained in the chapter below:

- *Boosted mood*

You might not know this but when you engage in healthy habits like working out and eating healthy, you do not only improve your body's health but you also improve your mental health.

Let me break it down for you; when you engage in physical activities, your body is usually stimulated to produce endorphins. Endorphins are chemicals which are produced in your brain and their main aim is to give you a happy feeling and make you feel relaxed. So by eating healthy and exercising, you also get to gain a joyous mood, which can be relaxing. An improved mood also helps you turn a negative day into a positive one because your head is inclined to think more positive. Who wouldn't want that?

- *Prevention of diseases*

The number one risk factor for diseases like heart diseases, stroke, cancer and osteoporosis is usually weight gain that leads to obesity. When you are obese from eating unhealthy foods, you usually attract osteoporosis.

Osteoporosis is a disease which is caused by lack of calcium which makes your bones weak and forces your organs to overwork.

Weight gain is also known for attracting high blood pressure and other cardiovascular diseases, which occur as a result of too much intake of saturated fats that leads to high cholesterol that builds up in your blood vessels.

When you eat healthy meals and work out, you automatically protect your body from a wide range of diseases. This is because healthy eating boosts the functionality of all of your organs. When your organs are 100% efficient, it is very hard for you to be attacked by diseases because the cells that protect you become much stronger and efficient in their work. Eating healthy also eliminates foods that cause diseases in your body like excessive fats. On the other hand, working out helps you to burn fat, which unblocks your vessels from cholesterol, which is something that reduces your chances of getting cardiovascular diseases.

- *Increase your life span*

In the world today, doctors have managed to discover surgical procedures that can make you look good on the outside. What they have been unable to come up with is a procedure that can add some years to your life. But that should never worry you because you don't need such kind of a procedure. What you need is a healthy diet and some exercises if you want your years to increase.

A certain study was carried out by The American Council on exercise. This study looked into the lives of 13,000 people where their physical activities were monitored over an eight year period. At the end of the study, the researchers found out that the people who used to walk for 30 minutes each and every day had reduced their chances of dying prematurely as compared to the their counterparts who didn't exercise occasionally.

According to that study, exercising can actually increase your lifespan and it can get even better if you are to combine exercising with healthy eating as your energy will be boosted to work out more.

- *Increases your body energy*

The other thing that you get to gain from following a healthy diet and working out is an increased energy in your body. Let me explain to you in a simpler way. Have you ever experienced a lethargic feeling that happened just after you ate your meal? That feeling is usually brought by eating unhealthy and an imbalanced meal; the kind of meal that can't provide your body with the energy it needs. By eating healthy balanced meals, your body usually gets the energy it needs to carry out and maintain its functions. That is why after eating healthy meals, you don't feel down and lazy; instead, you get an energetic and active feeling.

Regular exercises also increase your body's energy. It does that by delivering nutrients and oxygen into your tissues. That then makes your cardiovascular system start working in a more efficient manner, which results into you getting more energy. According to Mayo clinic, exercising also increases your muscle strength, which elevates your endurance as it provides your muscles with more energy.

Now you have seen why the subject of health and fitness is important to you. You have also seen the benefits that you stand to gain if you follow a healthy and fit lifestyle. So the next step for you is to learn how you can start living a healthy and fit life. All of that is going to be explained in the chapter below. So read on to gain more knowledge on this interesting topic of health and fitness.

How To Get Started

Getting fit and healthy is usually a dream come true for everyone. This is because attaining it improves the functionality of your body, which is something that we all welcome with open arms. Sadly, a very small percentage of people who try to get fit and healthy actually manage to achieve it. This is because people do not take their time to educate themselves on how to go about acquiring optimum health and fitness. This might come as a surprise to you but being healthy and fit takes more than just exercising and eating healthy. It requires planning and a high level of preparedness for what you are about to do to get optimum health and fitness.

In this chapter, you are going to learn about the first steps that you will need to take before you can jump into exercising or practicing healthy dieting. Check out these steps below.

Step 1: Set a Goal

Majority of people who fail to achieve optimum health and fitness usually have one thing in common; they don't sit down and determine why they want to achieve optimum health and fitness. In simple terms, they don't have a goal. Lack of a goal usually makes it easier for you to fall of the bandwagon when things get tough. This is because you do not have a burning reason why you are doing what you are doing.

So the first step that you will need to take in your journey to optimum health and fitness is to come up with a goal. But how are you supposed to do that? It's simple; you need to ask yourself what being healthy and fit means to you. Does it mean that you will now be able to run without going out of breath? Does it mean you will fit in your wedding clothes? Or does it mean you will be able to leave a more energetic and satisfying life?

You should come up with a reason that is personal and very dear to you. Reasons that can make do just about anything to achieve them. For example, your reason can be to lose weight in order to reduce your health problems.

Once you get a reason, the next step is for you to break it down so that it can be specific, measurable, attainable, realistic and timely. For example you can say, "My goal is to reduce my weight by 40 pounds in a period of 6 months so that I can break free from the danger of getting a heart attack as well as acquire a body which is energetic." That kind of goal will easily motivate you and keep you focused.

Step 2: Create A Visible Vision For Your Goal

Once you have your goal, the next step is for you to actually write in down and create a visual of the outcome that you desire. This is because it is easy for your brain to relate to a visual goal than thoughts, which can be just a wishful thinking for you. That's why you need to write down your goals and create a visual picture of your desired outcome in order to communicate to your mind that you are serious about a certain goal. For example, if you want to lose weight and gain an athletic body, you can stick a picture of a bodybuilder in your room so that your mind can constantly be reminded of what you want to achieve. This step is usually very important because it serves as a motivation in your journey to optimum health.

Step 3: Surround Yourself With Supportive People

The third step that you should take is to surround yourself with people who are striving for better health and fitness. By doing so, you create an atmosphere where you can be motivated and inspired to do better by the people around you.

To find a supportive group of people, you can start by searching for a community club in your area that meets for workouts or for healthy cooking lessons. The other thing that you can do to find a group of people who have the same passion and goal as yours is to look for seminars, which talk about healthy eating and working out. As the Bible says, "Iron sharpens iron." In simple terms, like-minded people improve and encourage each other and that is something that you need right now.

The above step by step preparation formula should be very important to you because it will greatly determine whether you will succeed or not. Therefore, you need to take them seriously by doing exactly what they have instructed you to do. Therefore, sit down and start figuring out what your goal is, write it down, create a visual of what you want to achieve and start looking for supportive groups before moving to the next step.

Once you're done with all that, you will now be ready to head on to the next step, which is learning what exercises you need to do to be fit. Check this out below.

The Best Training Program

Now that you have learnt the steps to take before you can give healthy living and fitness a shot, it's time to get down to business. By this, I mean it's time for you to learn what to do in order to achieve optimum health and fitness.

Basically, there are two things that you can do to be healthy and fit. One of them is to change your eating lifestyle to a healthy one and the second one is to start exercising and making your body fit and better.

In this guide, you will be educated on how to do the both of them. With that being said, this chapter is going to first focus on educating you on how to get fit through exercising.

Have you ever found it hard to climb up a stairs because you keep on going out of breath? Do you often have a constant lazy feeling that makes you uninspired to be active? And have you ever felt like you are too heavy and inflexible for your own liking? If your answer to the above questions is 'yes' then you are physically unfit and you need to exercise.

With that being said, it's difficult for you not to wonder where to start considering how complex working out is. But don't be worried; I am going to explain to you where to start and what to do next.

Exercising to achieve optimum health is a subject that is divided into two sections. The first section is you learning what types of exercises are ideal for you and the second section is a training program that will guide you on which exercises you need to do to achieve optimum fitness. Below is a breakdown of the two sections.

What Types Of Exercises Are Ideal For Optimum Fitness?

Basically, there are two types of exercises, which are ideal for optimum fitness. These exercises include; cardiovascular exercises, which includes cardio and aerobic and weight lifting or strength training exercises, which include resistance training. Let's break them down below;

Cardiovascular Exercises

Cardiovascular exercises are simply exercises that raise your heart rate. These exercises mostly work your muscles, including your heart, by using large muscle movements. The benefit of cardiovascular exercises comes from the muscle movements, which influence your capillaries to deliver more oxygen to your muscle cells and enables your body to burn more fat during and after exercising.

What that does to you is that it significantly reduces your weight, increases your energy levels and reduces your stress levels. Good examples of cardiovascular exercises include running, cycling and aerobics.

With that being said, cardio exercises do not give you a 6 pack or an increased muscle mass. It only makes your muscles stronger and increases the efficiency of your body together with improving your health, which is very important when carrying out your day to day activities.

Strength Training

Strength training is composed of exercises, which use resistance as a way of inducing muscle contractions. If you want to have a masculine body, then you are going to love strength training because strength training exercises will build your strength, endurance and the size of your muscles.

The main purpose of strength training is usually to improve your overall health and well-being through; the improvement of your joint function, the increase of your bone and the strength and toughness of your ligament. Examples of strength training exercises include body weight exercises like push-ups and squats, weight lifting exercises like barbell squats and barbell straight leg lifts and resistance bands exercises.

For you to attain optimum fitness and body health, you will need to combine the two types of exercise above. By performing both cardio and strength training exercises, you will be able to build muscles and a better body shape at the same time.

So how are you supposed to perform the two? The answer is simple; you need a workout plan, which will guide you on what to do and when to do it. Here is a guideline on what to do when:

The Best Training Program

Everyone in this universe has a different fitness level. What might work for you might not work for someone else and vice versa. With that in mind, I know you might still be wondering; how can you find the best training program for you? The answer is that you will need to learn the elements that make a good training program and then use them to custom make your own training program. So what elements are these? Check them out below:

- *Determine your situation*

The first element that you will need to look at when you want to come up with a training program is determining how much time you can devote to exercising each day. This is usually a very important element because there is no way you can benefit from a one hour per day exercising schedule by doing only 30 minutes of it.

Therefore, the first thing you can do is to figure out how much time you are willing to commit to exercising and then you will now be able to develop the most proficient workout within that time frame.

- *The type of exercises to do*

As you saw earlier, the ideal exercises for optimum health consist of cardiovascular exercises and strength training exercises. When making a good training program, you must make sure that the two exercises give you a full body routine by the end of the week.

What I mean by this is that you need to come up with a weekly routine that has at least one exercise for your core (abs and lower back), pull (forearms, biceps and back), push (triceps, shoulders and chest), quads and butt and hamstrings.

Having a well rounded routine helps you to develop a body shape that has been balanced muscle wise. Being masculine in only one or a few parts of your body will make you look ridiculous and you don't want that.

- *Warm up exercises*

A good training program must consist of a warm up exercise. Warm ups are usually exercises that you do to prepare your body for a workout. They (warm ups) are important because they protect your body from injuries like hamstrings strains. They do this by warming up your muscles as well as loosening up your joints to increase blood flow in your muscles.

Warm ups consists of light cardio and stretching exercises that are supposed to last for 5-10 minutes.

- *Cooling down exercises*

A good training program also needs a cooling down exercise, which is an exercise that you do after a workout. Cooling down exercises are normally very important because they give your muscles a chance to relax and also protect your body from undergoing a rapid drop of blood pressure, which can make you faint.

- *How long to rest between sets*

For you to make the most out of a training program, you need to know the ideal resting times in between sets. Resting time impacts the result of your work out because taking a long rest makes you lose the intensity in your workouts and too little of a rest in between sets makes you burn out quickly. Below is a guideline on the resting time that you will need to take.

✓ When doing 1-3 reps, you should rest for 3-5 minutes

✓ When doing 4-7 reps, rest for 2-3 minutes

✓ When doing 8-12 reps, rest for 1-2 minutes

✓ When doing more than 13 reps, rest for a minute or less.

Knowing the five elements of a good training program is important because it can help you create your own training program and also gives you knowledge on how to alter an already made training program to suit your needs.

With that being said, today you are not going to make your own training program because you are going to be provided with an all round training program for three weeks, which is amazing. Check it out below.

3 Weeks Training Program

Week 1

In the first week, you are going to take it slow by doing a 20 minutes workout each day. In every workout, you will need to start with a 5 minute warm up and finish with a 5 minute warm down.

The best warm up for you to do includes power walking, jumping jacks, jumping ropes, jogging, martial arts kicks and overhead arm circles.

The best warm down for you to do is light stretching each part of your body for about 5-10 seconds after a workout. Stretch the body parts that the exercise concentrated on more.

Monday- *Cardio exercises for thighs*

Run for 3 minutes and walk for 2 minutes. Repeat this 2 times.

Tuesday- *Core strength training*

✓ Planks: 3 sets of 10 reps. (30 seconds rest)

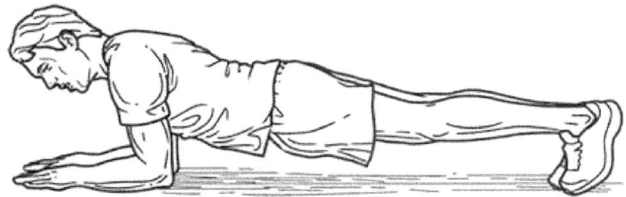

✓ Supermen pose: 3 sets of 10 reps (30 seconds rest)

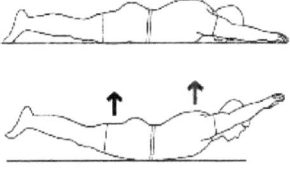

✓ Crunches: 3 sets of 10 reps (30 seconds resting time)

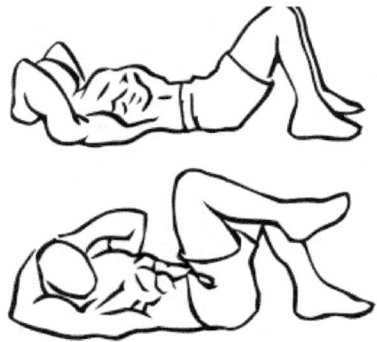

Wednesday- *cardio exercises for the arms*

- ✓ Jumping rope: 2 sets of 10 reps (30 seconds rest)

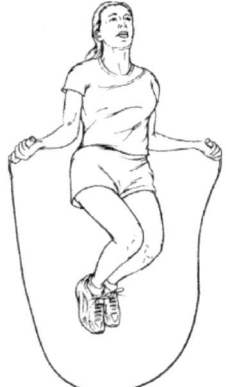

- ✓ Push-ups: 2 sets of 10 reps (30 seconds rest)

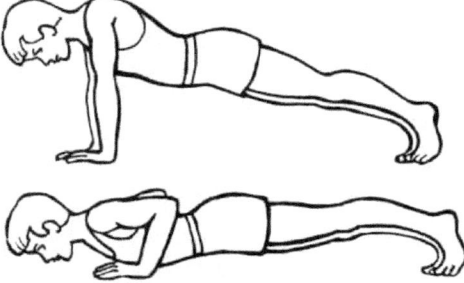

- ✓ Plank slaps: 2 sets of 5 reps (45 minutes rest)

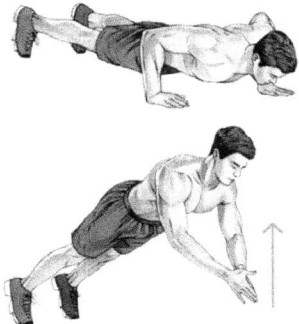

Thursday- *Butt and hamstring exercises*

✓ Step-up: 2 sets of 10 reps (30 seconds resting time)

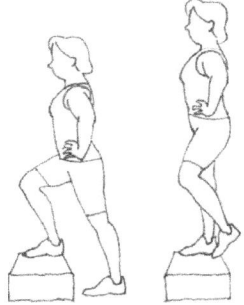

✓ Hip thrust: 2 sets of 10 reps (30 seconds resting time)

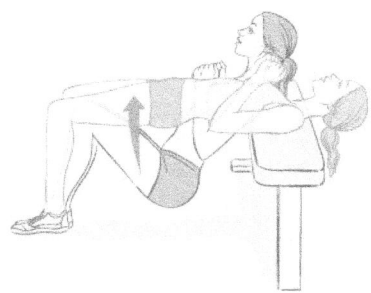

✓ Barbell squat: 2 sets of 10 reps (45 minutes resting time)

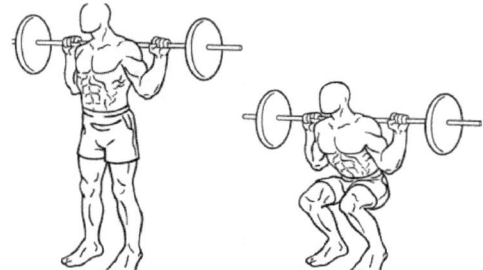

Friday- *cardio exercises for the shoulders*

✓ Overhead medicine ball slam: 2 sets of 10 reps (45 seconds rest)

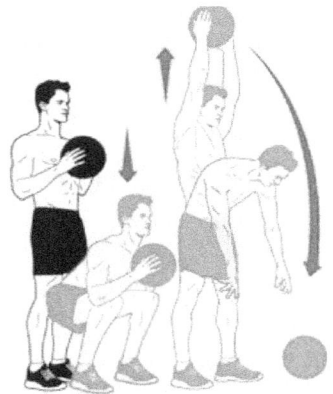

✓ Burpees: 2 sets of 10 reps (30 seconds rest)

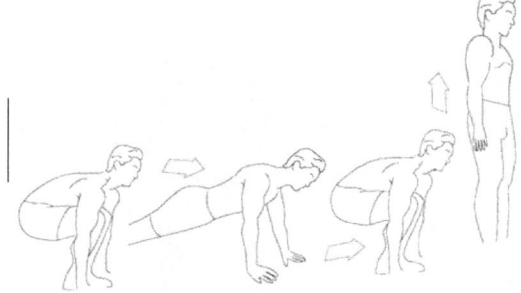

✓ Dumbbell upright row. 2 sets of 10 reps (30 seconds rest)

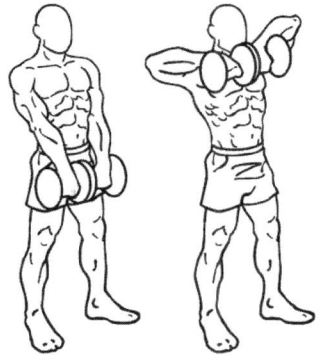

Saturday and Sunday

Rest

Week 2

In the second week, you are going to increase the intensity of your workouts by increasing the exercising time from 20 minutes to 30 minutes per session. Remember the first 5 minutes of your day's workout should consist of a warm up and the last 5 minutes a warm down.

Monday- *Cardio exercise for the whole body*

✓ Run for 4 minutes and walk for 1 minute. Repeat this 4 times.

Tuesday- *Core strength training*

✓ Seated barbell twist: 3 sets of 12 reps each (30 seconds rest)

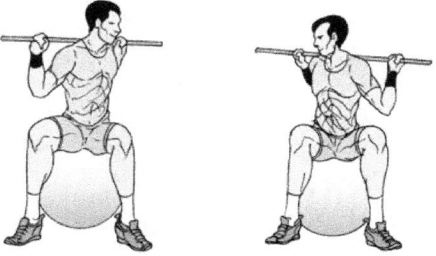

✓ Air bike: 3 sets 15 reps (30 seconds rest)

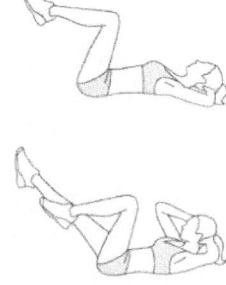

✓ Cable crunch. 3 sets 15 reps (45 seconds rest)

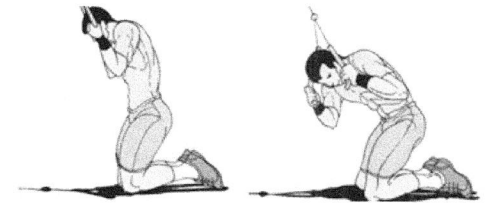

Wednesday- *Cardio exercises for the back*

✓ Bend over rows: 3 sets of 15 reps (30 seconds rest)

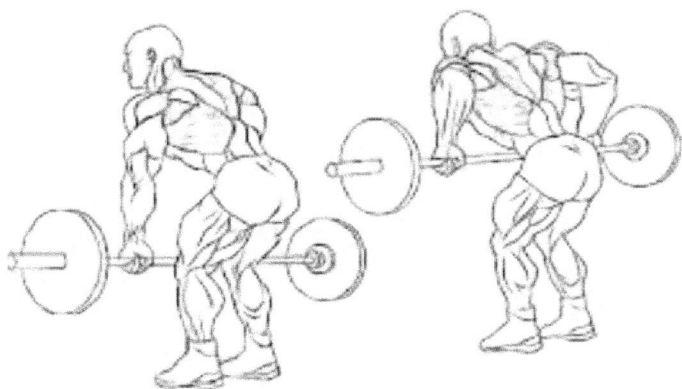

✓ Lat pull-downs: 3 sets of 15 reps (30 seconds rest)

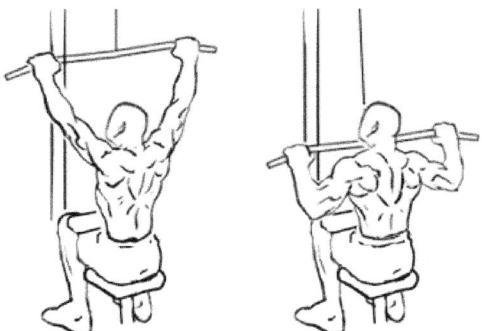

✓ Roman chair back extension: 3 sets of 15 reps (30 second rest)

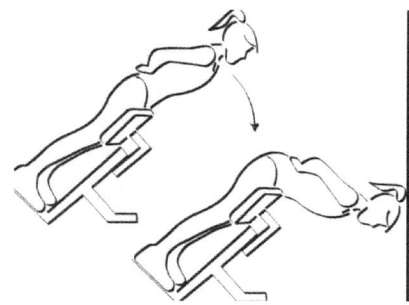

Thursday- *pull strength training*

✓ Chin ups: 3 sets of 15 reps (30 seconds resting time)

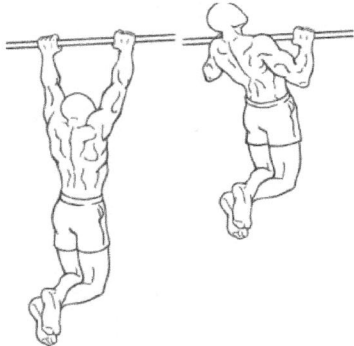

Dumbbell alternate bicep curl: 3 sets of 15 reps (30 seconds rest)

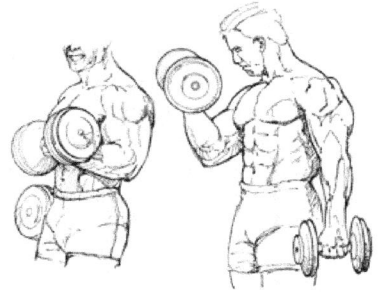

✓ Finger curls: 3 sets of 15 reps (30 seconds rest)

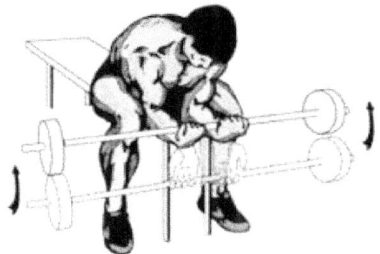

Friday- *cardio for shoulders, triceps and chest*

✓ Chest-fly: 3 sets of 12 reps (40 seconds rest)

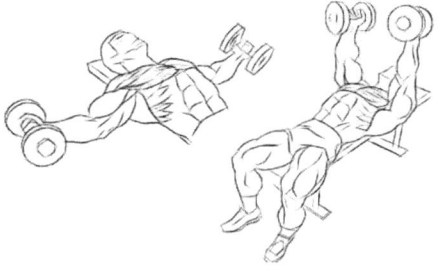

✓ Bent over triceps extensions:3 sets of 12 reps (40 seconds rest)

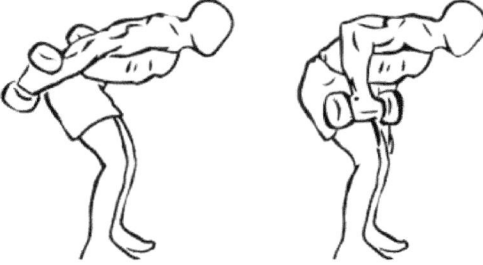

✓ Dumbbell pullover: 3 sets of 12 reps (40 seconds rest)

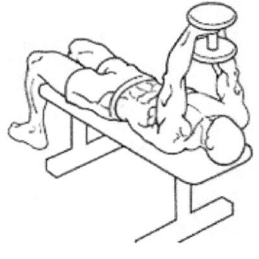 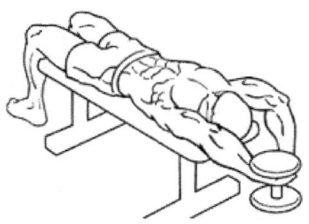

Saturday and Sunday

Rest

Week 3

By now, your body should be used to exercising regularly. So in this week, you are going to move to advanced exercises and add an additional 10 minutes for exercising. So now you will be exercising for 40 minutes.

Monday- *cardio exercises*

✓ Run for 8 minutes and walk for 2 minutes. Repeat this 3 times

Tuesday- *core strength training*

✓ Reverse crunch: 3 sets 15 reps (30 seconds rest)

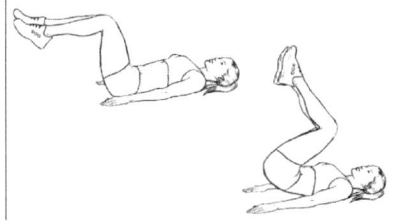

✓ Exercise ball crunch: 3 sets for 15 reps (30 seconds rest)

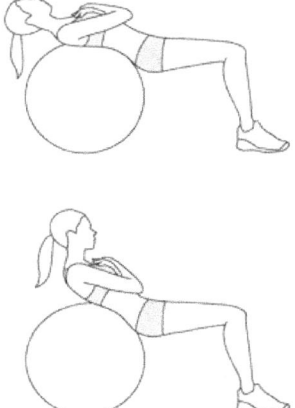

✓ Decline crunch: 3 sets for 12 reps (40 seconds rest)

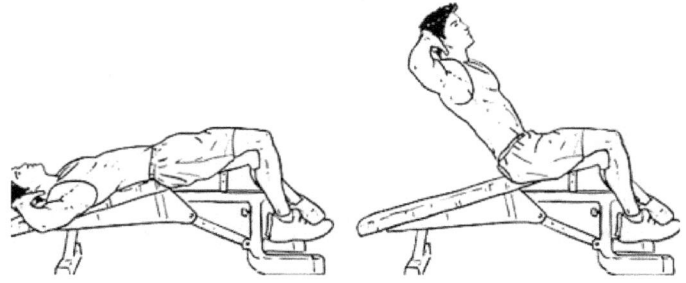

✓ Frog sit-ups. 3 sets for 15 reps (30 seconds rest)

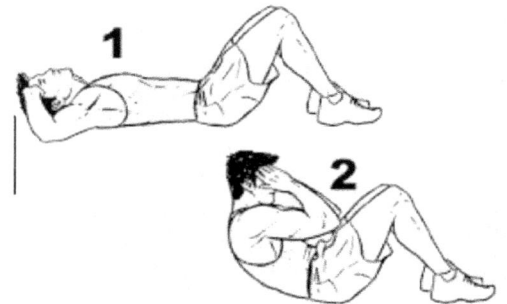

Wednesday- *cardio exercises for butt and hamstring*

✓ Goblet squat: 3 sets of 12 reps (30 seconds rest)

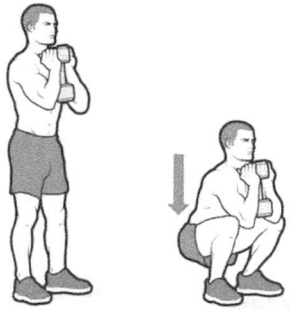

- Lunge with biceps curl. 3 sets of 12 reps (30 seconds rest)

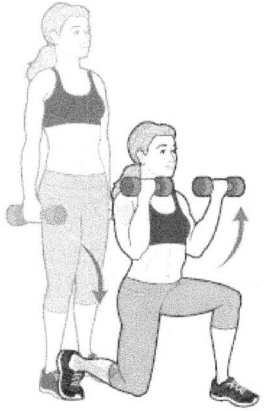

✓ Box jump: 3 sets of 10 reps (30 seconds rest)

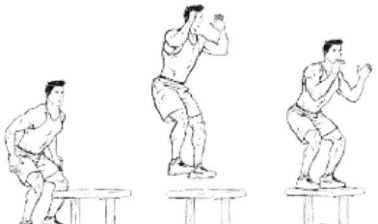

✓ Burpees: 3 sets of 10 reps (30 seconds rest)

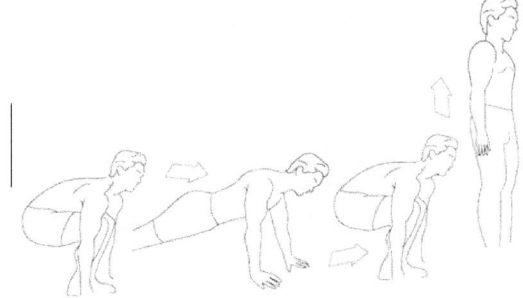

Thursday- *pull strength training*

✓ Straight bar cable curls: 3 sets of 10 reps (30 seconds rest)

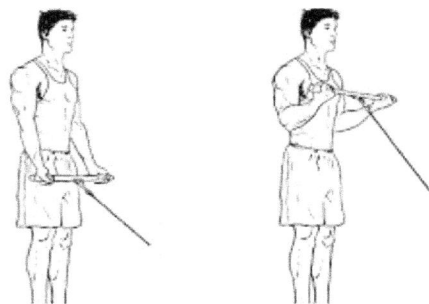

✓ Barbell-reverse curls: 3 sets of 10 reps (40 seconds rest)

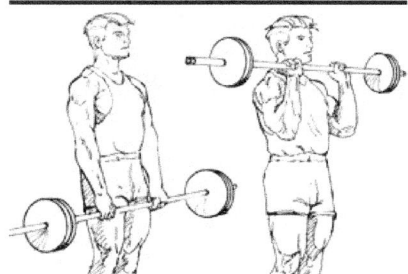

✓ Reverse cable curls: 3 sets of 10 reps (40 seconds rest)

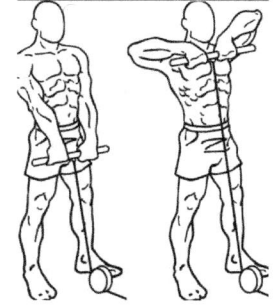

✓ Seated cable row: 3 sets of 10 reps (40 seconds rest)

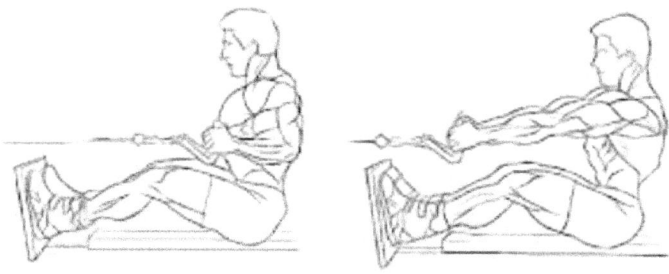

Friday- *push cardio exercises*

✓ Incline press: 3 sets of 10 reps (30 seconds rest)

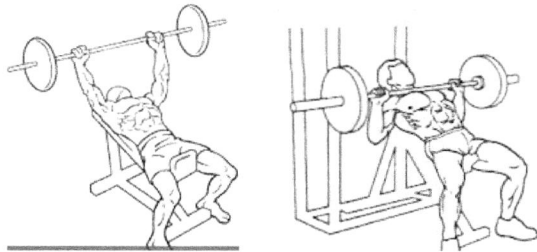

✓ Close-grip press: 3 sets of 10 reps (30 seconds rest)

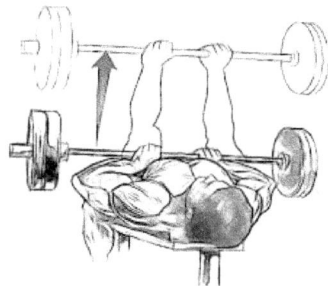

✓ Triceps lift: 3 sets of 15 reps (30 seconds rest)

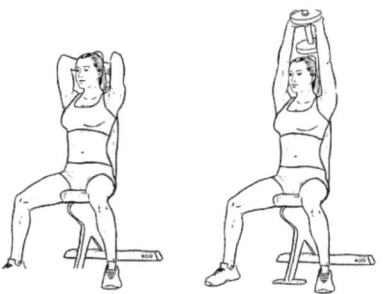

- Military press. 3 sets of 15 reps (30 seconds rest)

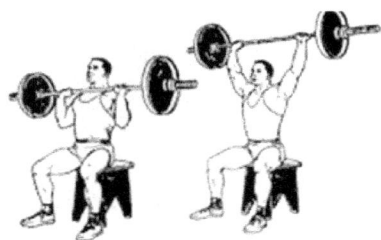

Saturday and Sunday

Rest

What you have just seen above is one of the best training programs that you can use to make yourself more masculine, energetic, healthy and physically fit. As I said earlier, what may work for me, may not work for you so feel free to readjust the training program to fit your time schedule and ability. For example, if you find that you have too much time on your hands, you can increase the working out time by increasing the sets of the exercises. But if you have limited time for exercising then you can reduce the sets. If you also find that a workout is too difficult for you, you can reduce the reps or the sets to that workout first.

Remember the idea here is for you to be physically fit so don't try and compete to do what your body is not comfortable with. Instead, take your own time and go with your own pace.

With that being said, you can never achieve optimum health and fitness by only exercising. You need to combine it with a healthy eating lifestyle and that brings us to our next chapter.

30 Day's Food For A Healthy Body

As you have seen above, exercising and healthy eating go hand in hand; one cannot do without the other, as each of them is equally important to your overall health and fitness. So now that you know how to work out and you even have a training program to follow, the next step for you is to learn healthy eating patterns that will keep your body healthy.

At the beginning of this book, we saw that thousands of years ago, the world was very different from what it is today. One of the notable differences was in the food that was eaten back then and the food that is being eaten today. Back then, our ancestors used to eat natural foods like vegetables, meat, roots, and fruits, which they got them from hunting and gathering ,which is unlike the today's world where we eat processed and manufactured foods, which are full of additives and chemicals. Back then, our ancestors didn't experience some of the terminal diseases we have today and they were healthy and physically fit.

According to the above summary, it is common sense that the only way for you to be healthy is by going back to your roots and eating what your forefathers used to eat.

So what did our forefathers eat exactly? Below is a summary of what they ate and what we should eat:

✓ **Fruits**- they ate both fresh and dried fruits

✓ **Vegetables**- they ate all types of vegetables.

✓ **Meat**- they ate all types of meat and poultry like ducks, turkeys, beef, pork, lambs and wild animals. Organic, grass fed, wild etc.

✓ **Nuts and seeds**. They ate all types of seeds excluding peanuts which are legumes.

✓ **Fish and sea foods**- like lobsters, scallops, shrimp and crabs.

✓ **Some fats**- like ghee, coconut oils, plant oils and duck fat.

Note: The above were organic and all natural without any additives, chemicals or 'human' intervention.

Some of the foods that they didn't have and we need to avoid include:

- ✓ **Artificial sweeteners and sugar-** like agave syrup, maple syrup, honey and raw sugar

- ✓ **All types of alcohol-** including wines, spirits and beer

- ✓ **Dairy products-** like ice cream, milk, yoghurt and cheese.

- ✓ **Soy products-** like soy sauce and miso

- ✓ **All types of grains-** like rice, oats and corn.

- ✓ **Legumes and pulses** – like snow peas, green beans, peanut butter, lentils and beans

- ✓ **Food additives** – like sulfites and carrageenan.

If you want to adapt to a healthy life, you will have to adhere to the two lists above. By this, I mean you need to practice eating what is allowed in the above list and ignore what is prohibited.

With that being said, it is not enough to just eat what is allowed and ignore what is not. You need a meal plan, which will discipline and organize your healthy eating lifestyle by outlining what you need to eat for your breakfast, lunch and dinner.

Below is one of the best meal plans that you can follow to achieve optimum health.

30 Day's Healthy Food Plan

Week 1

Breakfast

- ✓ Easy egg omelet that you can cook with vegetables filling.
- ✓ A paleo pancake that comprises of a combination of bananas, eggs and almond butter.
- ✓ A cinnamon, butternut and date smoothie
- ✓ Sweet potato breakfast skillet with a combination of bacon

Lunch

- ✓ Frittata that is made of asparagus and smoked salmon
- ✓ Egg muffins with raw veggies
- ✓ Grilled fish with sweet potato mash and a topping of salsa
- ✓ Chicken shawarma salad

Dinner

- ✓ A stew made with mushrooms, onions, squash and beef
- ✓ Sweet and sour pork chops
- ✓ Cauliflower crust pizza
- ✓ Mahi-mahi fish tacos. Grilled

Week 2

Breakfast

- ✓ Portobello breakfast sandwich with bacon and avocado
- ✓ Blueberry muffin that uses almond flour
- ✓ Bread French toast that is made with banana.
- ✓ Vegetable salad with eggs

Lunch

- ✓ Baked zucchini halves that are stuffed with tomato sauce and ground beef

- ✓ Lettuce wrapped with tuna
- ✓ Chicken soup with kale
- ✓ Fried chicken fingers

Dinner

- ✓ Meat and spaghetti squash lasagna
- ✓ Paleo egg rolls
- ✓ Baked Italian meatballs with marinara sauce
- ✓ Roasted chicken that is served with vegetables and cranberries

Week 3

Breakfast

- ✓ Green smoothie made out of bananas, spinach and avocado
- ✓ Sweet potato waffles that are made from almond and coconut flours
- ✓ Fried eggs and a veggie sandwich
- ✓ Raspberry sherbet Chia pudding

Lunch

- ✓ Sauerkraut hot dog buns
- ✓ Lemon tuna bowl
- ✓ Soup that comprises of homemade meatballs and kale
- ✓ Thai basil beef

Dinner

- ✓ Shredded chicken enchilada guacamole burgers
- ✓ Sweet lemon shrimp
- ✓ Creamy basil with tomato chicken
- ✓ Duck and vegetables

Week 4

Breakfast

✓ A smoothie that is made from parsley, bananas, avocado and apples

✓ Stuffed avocados which comprise of red peppers, shrimp and crabs

✓ Sweet potato hash browns

✓ Meat bagels which consist of beef stuffed with vegetables.

Lunch

✓ Avocado egg salad

✓ Supreme pizza frittata

✓ Zucchini patties with some salad on the side

✓ Ground pork and some cabbage.

Dinner

✓ Stuffed mushroom that consists of tomato, avocado, meatballs and alfalfa sprouts.

✓ Zucchini beef skillet

✓ Lemon shrimp

✓ Tuna and tomato burgers.

By following the above meal plan, you will have eliminated all those manufactured and processed foods from your menu, which bring nothing to you but diseases and an unhealthy body. Eating the meals above will be like a breath of fresh air to your health.

Conclusion

We have come to the end of the book. Thank you for reading and congratulations for reading until the end.

I hope you have found the book helpful and eye opening.

The thing is; your health is the most important thing in your life. It's what keeps you going. By following all the instructions that you have been given in this book, you will be able to improve your health and at the same time develop a better looking body. So don't waste any more time being unhealthy; start following the training program and the meal plan today.

If you found the book valuable, can you recommend it to others? One way to do that is to post a review on Amazon.

Click here to leave a review for this book on Amazon!

Thank you and good luck!

www.ingramcontent.com/pod-product-compliance
Lightning Source LLC
Chambersburg PA
CBHW062029280526
45787CB00005B/2263